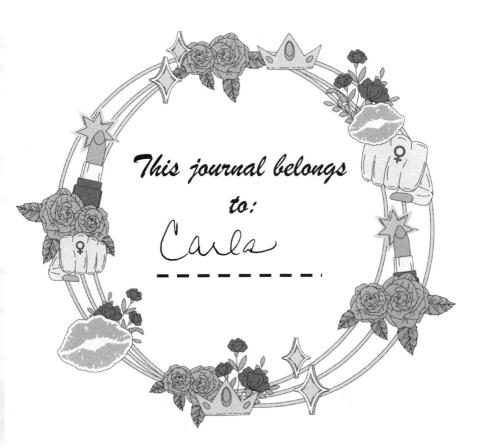

This journal belongs to:

Carla

My Daily Appointments

6 a.m.

7 a.m.

8 a.m.

9 a.m.

10 a.m.

11 a.m.

12 p.m.

1 p.m.

2 p.m.

3 p.m.

4 p.m.

5 p.m.

6 p.m.

7 p.m.

8 p.m.

9 p.m.

Medical Appointments

MEDICAL RECORDS FOR:

DOCTORS OFFICE:

DATE:	DESCRIPTION:	NEXT APPOINTMENT:

Medical Checkups

MONTH:

MONTH:

MONTH:

MONTH:

MONTH:

MONTH:

MONTH:

MONTH:

MONTH:

MONTH:

MONTH:

MONTH:

Specialist Visits

DATE:

FOLLOW UP:

DOCTOR:

HOSPITAL:

REASON/PURPOSE:

NOTES:

DATE:

FOLLOW UP:

DOCTOR:

HOSPITAL:

REASON/PURPOSE:

NOTES:

Doctor Visits

NAME:

DATE:	DOCTOR:	REASON:	RESULTS:

Medications

NAME: _____   MONTH: _____

MEDICATION:	USED FOR:	DOSE:	TIMES PER DAY:

Surgeries

NAME: **DATE:**

DATE:	DOCTOR:	REASON:	RESULTS:

Treatments

NAME:

DATE:	TYPE:	PURPOSE:	DOCTOR:

Test Results

PERIOD OF:

DATE:	TEST:	DOCTOR:	PURPOSE:	RESULTS

Illness Tracker

DATE:	DESCRIPTION:	DR. VISIT	TREATMENT
		☐	☐
		☐	☐
		☐	☐
		☐	☐
		☐	☐
		☐	☐
		☐	☐
		☐	☐
		☐	☐
		☐	☐
		☐	☐
		☐	☐
		☐	☐
		☐	☐
		☐	☐
		☐	☐
		☐	☐
		☐	☐
		☐	☐
		☐	☐
		☐	☐
		☐	☐
		☐	☐

Symptom Tracker

DATE:	DESCRIPTION:	DR. VISIT	TREATMENT
		☐	☐
		☐	☐
		☐	☐
		☐	☐
		☐	☐
		☐	☐
		☐	☐
		☐	☐
		☐	☐
		☐	☐
		☐	☐
		☐	☐
		☐	☐
		☐	☐
		☐	☐
		☐	☐
		☐	☐
		☐	☐
		☐	☐
		☐	☐
		☐	☐
		☐	☐

Monthly Health Tracker

JANUARY	FEBRUARY	MARCH

APRIL	MAY	JUNE

Monthly Health Tracker

JULY	AUGUST	SEPTEMBER

OCTOBER	NOVEMBER	DECEMBER

Yearly Health Tracker

YEAR: ....

JANUARY	FEBRUARY	MARCH

APRIL	MAY	JUNE

JULY	AUGUST	SEPTEMBER

OCTOBER	NOVEMBER	DECEMBER

NOTES:

My Medical History

NAME: BIRTH DATE:

FAMILY DOCTOR: CONTACT:

BLOOD TYPE:

MEDICATIONS:

ALLERGIES:

DATE:	TREATMENTS, SURGERIES:	NOTES:

Medical Contacts

FAMILY DOCTOR

NAME:

ADDRESS:

PHONE:

ADDITIONAL INFO:

ONCOLOGIST

NAME:

ADDRESS:

PHONE:

ADDITIONAL INFO:

SPECIALIST

NAME:

ADDRESS:

PHONE:

ADDITIONAL INFO:

DENTIST

NAME:

ADDRESS:

PHONE:

ADDITIONAL INFO:

OTHER

NAME:

ADDRESS:

PHONE:

ADDITIONAL INFO:

Medical Expenses

YEAR:

DATE:	DESCRIPTION:	INSURANCE %:	COST:

My Medical Notes

A Girl Need's Goals

YEAR: ....

JANUARY

FEBRUARY

MARCH

APRIL

MAY

JUNE

JULY

AUGUST

SEPTEMBER

OCTOBER

NOVEMBER

DECEMBER

NOTES:

Take A Break & Doodle

Time To Doodle

My Goals For This Month

Month _____

Describe Your Goal

_____
_____
_____
_____

Why I Want to Achieve This Goal

_____
_____
_____

Steps I Will Take To Achieve My Goal

1. _____

2. _____

3. _____

4. _____

Motivation Keeps Me Movin'

DON'T FORGET TO *love yourself*

My motivation for this month is:

_____

_____

I want to work on this because:

_____

_____

_____

_____

Reflections

_____

_____

_____

_____

_____

_____

_____

_____

Today's
Affirmation

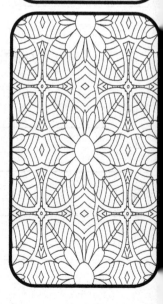

Empowering Quote Of The Week

Quote of the week:

What I will do for me this week...

To Do List

- ☐
- ☐
- ☐
- ☐
- ☐
- ☐

Thoughts....

Empowering Quote Of The Week

Quote of the week:

Thoughts....

What I will do for me this week...

To Do List

- ☐
- ☐
- ☐
- ☐
- ☐
- ☐

Empowering Quote Of The Week

Quote of the week:

What I will do for me this week...

To Do List

- ☐
- ☐
- ☐
- ☐
- ☐
- ☐

Thoughts....

Empowering Quote Of The Week

Quote of the week:

What I will do for me this week...

To Do List

- ☐
- ☐
- ☐
- ☐
- ☐
- ☐

Thoughts....

Monthly Prompts

Monthly Gratitude
List what you are grateful for this month.

_____
_____
_____
_____
_____
_____
_____

I am Learning…
What are you learning this month?

_____
_____
_____
_____
_____
_____
_____

People in my Life
Who are you grateful for today and why?

_____
_____
_____
_____
_____
_____
_____

Reflection
Write about the best part of your month.

_____
_____
_____
_____
_____
_____

Best Times of This Month

Date:
_____

What I saw:

Things I heard:

What I tasted:

My Feelings:

My Choices:

My Actions:

My Goals:

Overall thoughts of the month:

My Goals For This Month

Month _____

Describe Your Goal

_____

_____

_____

_____

Why I Want to Achieve This Goal

_____

_____

_____

Steps I Will Take To Achieve My Goal

1. _____

2. _____

3. _____

4. _____

Motivation Keeps Me Movin'

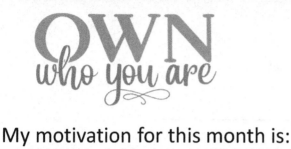

My motivation for this month is:

_____

_____

I want to work on this because:

_____

_____

_____

_____

Reflections

_____

_____

_____

_____

_____

_____

_____

Today's
Affirmation

Empowering Quote Of The Week

Quote of the week:

What I will do for me this week...

To Do List

- ☐
- ☐
- ☐
- ☐
- ☐
- ☐

Thoughts....

Empowering Quote Of The Week

Quote of the week:

What I will do for me this week...

To Do List

- ☐
- ☐
- ☐
- ☐
- ☐
- ☐

Thoughts....

Empowering Quote Of The Week

Quote of the week:

What I will do for me this week...

To Do List

- ☐
- ☐
- ☐
- ☐
- ☐
- ☐

Thoughts....

Empowering Quote Of The Week

Quote of the week:

What I will do for me this week...

To Do List

- ☐
- ☐
- ☐
- ☐
- ☐
- ☐

Thoughts....

Monthly Prompts

Monthly Gratitude
List what you are
grateful for this month.

_____
_____
_____
_____
_____
_____

I am Learning…
What are you learning
this month?

_____
_____
_____
_____
_____
_____

People in my Life
Who are you grateful for
today and why?

_____
_____
_____
_____
_____
_____

Reflection
Write about the best
part of your month.

_____
_____
_____
_____
_____
_____

Best Times of This Month

Date: _____

What I saw:

Things I heard:

What I tasted:

My Feelings:

My Choices:

My Actions:

My Goals:

Overall thoughts of the month:

My Goals For This Month

Month

Describe Your Goal

_____

_____

_____

_____

Why I Want to Achieve This Goal

_____

_____

_____

Steps I Will Take To Achieve My Goal

1. _____

2. _____

3. _____

4. _____

Motivation Keeps Me Movin'

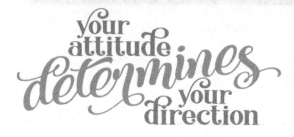
your attitude determines your direction

My motivation for this month is:

_____

_____

I want to work on this because:

_____

_____

_____

Reflections

_____

_____

_____

_____

_____

_____

_____

Today's Affirmation

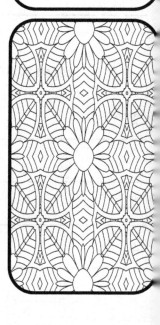

Empowering Quote Of The Week

Quote of the week:

What I will do for me this week...

To Do List

- ❑
- ❑
- ❑
- ❑
- ❑
- ❑

Thoughts....

Empowering Quote Of The Week

Quote of the week:

What I will do for me this week...

To Do List

- ☐
- ☐
- ☐
- ☐
- ☐
- ☐

Thoughts....

Empowering Quote Of The Week

Quote of the week:

Thoughts....

What I will do for me this week...

To Do List

- ☐
- ☐
- ☐
- ☐
- ☐
- ☐

Empowering Quote Of The Week

Quote of the week:

What I will do for me this week...

To Do List

- ☐
- ☐
- ☐
- ☐
- ☐
- ☐

Thoughts....

Monthly Prompts

Monthly Gratitude
List what you are
grateful for this month.

_____

_____

_____

_____

_____

_____

I am Learning...
What are you learning
this month?

_____

_____

_____

_____

_____

_____

People in my Life
Who are you grateful for
today and why?

_____

_____

_____

_____

_____

_____

_____

Reflection
Write about the best
part of your month.

_____

_____

_____

_____

_____

_____

Best Times of This Month

Date: _____

What I saw:

Things I heard:

What I tasted:

My Feelings:

My Choices:

My Actions:

My Goals:

Overall thoughts of the month:

My Goals For This Month

Month _____

Describe Your Goal

_____

_____

_____

_____

Why I Want to Achieve This Goal

_____

_____

_____

Steps I Will Take To Achieve My Goal

1. _____

2. _____

3. _____

4. _____

Whatever YOUR CREATIVE heart Desires

My motivation for this month is:

_____

_____

I want to work on this because:

_____

_____

_____

_____

Reflections

_____

_____

_____

_____

_____

_____

_____

Today's
Affirmation

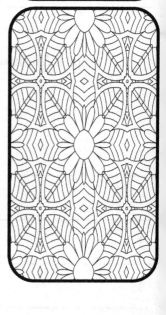

Empowering Quote Of The Week

Quote of the week:

What I will do for me this week...

To Do List

- ☐
- ☐
- ☐
- ☐
- ☐
- ☐

Thoughts....

Empowering Quote Of The Week

Quote of the week:

What I will do for me this week...

To Do List

- ☐
- ☐
- ☐
- ☐
- ☐
- ☐

Thoughts....

Empowering Quote Of The Week

Quote of the week:

What I will do for me this week...

To Do List

- ❑
- ❑
- ❑
- ❑
- ❑
- ❑

Thoughts....

Empowering Quote Of The Week

Quote of the week:

What I will do for me this week...

To Do List

- ☐
- ☐
- ☐
- ☐
- ☐
- ☐

Thoughts....

Monthly Prompts

Monthly Gratitude
List what you are
grateful for this month.

_____
_____
_____
_____
_____
_____

I am Learning...
What are you learning
this month?

_____
_____
_____
_____
_____
_____

People in my Life
Who are you grateful for
today and why?

_____
_____
_____
_____
_____
_____

Reflection
Write about the best
part of your month.

_____
_____
_____
_____
_____
_____

Best Times of This Month

Date: _____

What I saw:

Things I heard:

What I tasted:

My Feelings:

My Choices:

My Actions:

My Goals:

Overall thoughts of the month:

My Goals For This Month

Month _____

Describe Your Goal

_____

_____

_____

_____

Why I Want to Achieve This Goal

_____

_____

_____

Steps I Will Take To Achieve My Goal

1. _____

2. _____

3. _____

4. _____

Motivation Keeps Me Movin'

GET OUT OF your own way

My motivation for this month is:

_____

_____

I want to work on this because:

_____

_____

_____

_____

Reflections

_____

_____

_____

_____

_____

_____

_____

Today's
Affirmation

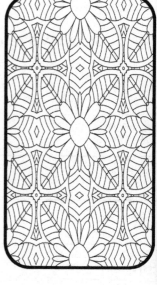

Empowering Quote Of The Week

Quote of the week:

What I will do for me this week...

To Do List

- ☐
- ☐
- ☐
- ☐
- ☐
- ☐

Thoughts....

Empowering Quote Of The Week

Quote of the week:

What I will do for me this week...

To Do List

- ☐
- ☐
- ☐
- ☐
- ☐
- ☐

Thoughts....

Empowering Quote Of The Week

Quote of the week:

What I will do for me this week...

To Do List

- ❑
- ❑
- ❑
- ❑
- ❑
- ❑

Thoughts....

Empowering Quote Of The Week

Quote of the week:

Thoughts....

What I will do for me this week...

To Do List

- ☐
- ☐
- ☐
- ☐
- ☐
- ☐

Monthly Prompts

Monthly Gratitude
List what you are
grateful for this month.

_____
_____
_____
_____
_____
_____

I am Learning…
What are you learning
this month?

_____
_____
_____
_____
_____
_____

People in my Life
Who are you grateful for
today and why?

_____
_____
_____
_____
_____
_____

Reflection
Write about the best
part of your month.

_____
_____
_____
_____
_____
_____

Best Times of This Month

Date:
_____

What I saw:

Things I heard:

What I tasted:

My Feelings:

My Choices:

My Actions:

My Goals:

Overall thoughts of the month:

My Goals For This Month

Month _____

Describe Your Goal

_____

_____

_____

_____

Why I Want to Achieve This Goal

_____

_____

_____

Steps I Will Take To Achieve My Goal

1. _____

2. _____

3. _____

4. _____

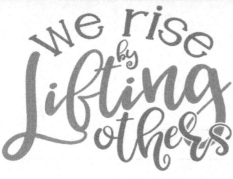

My motivation for this month is:

_____

_____

I want to work on this because:

_____

_____

_____

_____

Reflections

_____

_____

_____

_____

_____

_____

_____

Today's
Affirmation

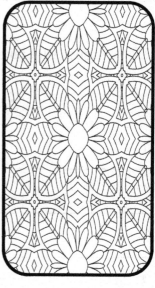

Empowering Quote Of The Week

Quote of the week:

What I will do for me this week...

To Do List

- ☐
- ☐
- ☐
- ☐
- ☐
- ☐

Thoughts....

Empowering Quote Of The Week

Quote of the week:

Thoughts....

What I will do for me this week...

To Do List

- ☐
- ☐
- ☐
- ☐
- ☐
- ☐

Empowering Quote Of The Week

Quote of the week:

What I will do for me this week...

To Do List

- ☐
- ☐
- ☐
- ☐
- ☐
- ☐

Thoughts....

Empowering Quote Of The Week

Quote of the week:

What I will do for me this week...

To Do List

- ☐
- ☐
- ☐
- ☐
- ☐
- ☐

Thoughts....

Monthly Prompts

Monthly Gratitude
List what you are grateful for this month.

_____
_____
_____
_____
_____
_____
_____

I am Learning...
What are you learning this month?

_____
_____
_____
_____
_____
_____
_____

People in my Life
Who are you grateful for today and why?

_____
_____
_____
_____
_____
_____
_____

Reflection
Write about the best part of your month.

_____
_____
_____
_____
_____
_____
_____

Best Times of This Month

Date:
_____

What I saw:

Things I heard:

What I tasted:

My Feelings:

My Choices:

My Actions:

My Goals:

Overall thoughts of the month:

My Goals For This Month

Month _____

Describe Your Goal

_____

_____

_____

_____

Why I Want to Achieve This Goal

_____

_____

Steps I Will Take To Achieve My Goal

1. _____

2. _____

3. _____

4. _____

DON'T BE AFRAID TO Sparkle A LITTLE BRIGHTER

My motivation for this month is:

_____
_____

I want to work on this because:

_____
_____
_____
_____

Reflections

_____
_____
_____
_____
_____
_____
_____
_____

Today's Affirmation

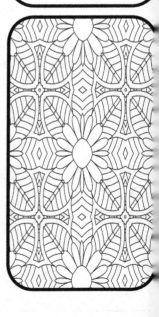

Empowering Quote Of The Week

Quote of the week:

What I will do for me this week...

To Do List

- ☐
- ☐
- ☐
- ☐
- ☐
- ☐

Thoughts....

Empowering Quote Of The Week

Quote of the week:

What I will do for me this week...

To Do List

- ☐
- ☐
- ☐
- ☐
- ☐
- ☐

Thoughts....

Empowering Quote Of The Week

Quote of the week:

What I will do for me this week...

To Do List

- ☐
- ☐
- ☐
- ☐
- ☐
- ☐

Thoughts....

Empowering Quote Of The Week

Quote of the week:

Thoughts....

What I will do for me this week...

To Do List

- ☐
- ☐
- ☐
- ☐
- ☐
- ☐

Monthly Prompts

Monthly Gratitude
List what you are grateful for this month.

_____
_____
_____
_____
_____
_____

I am Learning...
What are you learning this month?

_____
_____
_____
_____
_____
_____

People in my Life
Who are you grateful for today and why?

_____
_____
_____
_____
_____
_____

Reflection
Write about the best part of your month.

_____
_____
_____
_____
_____
_____

Best Times of This Month

Date:

_____

What I saw:

Things I heard:

What I tasted:

My Feelings:

My Choices:

My Actions:

My Goals:

Overall thoughts of the month:

My Goals For This Month

Month _____

Describe Your Goal

_____

_____

_____

_____

Why I Want to Achieve This Goal

_____

_____

_____

Steps I Will Take To Achieve My Goal

1. _____

2. _____

3. _____

4. _____

WHAT WOULD you do IF, YOU WEREN'T afraid

My motivation for this month is:
_____
_____

I want to work on this because:
_____
_____
_____
_____

Reflections
_____
_____
_____
_____
_____
_____
_____
_____

Today's
Affirmation

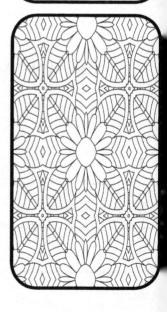

Empowering Quote Of The Week

Quote of the week:

What I will do for me this week...

To Do List

- ☐
- ☐
- ☐
- ☐
- ☐
- ☐

Thoughts....

Empowering Quote Of The Week

Quote of the week:

What I will do for me this week...

To Do List

- ☐
- ☐
- ☐
- ☐
- ☐
- ☐

Thoughts....

Empowering Quote Of The Week

Quote of the week:

What I will do for me this week...

To Do List

- ☐
- ☐
- ☐
- ☐
- ☐
- ☐

Thoughts....

Empowering Quote Of The Week

Quote of the week:

Thoughts….

What I will do for me this week...

To Do List

- ☐
- ☐
- ☐
- ☐
- ☐
- ☐

Monthly Prompts

Monthly Gratitude
List what you are
grateful for this month.

_____
_____
_____
_____
_____
_____
_____

I am Learning…
What are you learning
this month?

_____
_____
_____
_____
_____
_____
_____

People in my Life
Who are you grateful for
today and why?

_____
_____
_____
_____
_____
_____
_____

Reflection
Write about the best
part of your month.

_____
_____
_____
_____
_____
_____
_____

Best Times of This Month

Date:
_____

What I saw:

Things I heard:

What I tasted:

My Feelings:

My Choices:

My Actions:

My Goals:

Overall thoughts of the month:

My Goals For This Month

Month _____

Describe Your Goal

_____

_____

_____

_____

Why I Want to Achieve This Goal

_____

_____

_____

Steps I Will Take To Achieve My Goal

1. _____

2. _____

3. _____

4. _____

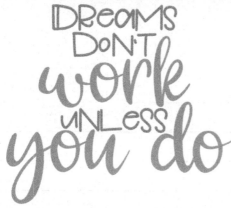

My motivation for this month is:

_____

_____

I want to work on this because:

_____

_____

_____

_____

Reflections

_____

_____

_____

_____

_____

_____

_____

_____

_____

Today's
Affirmation

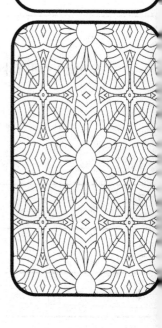

Empowering Quote Of The Week

Quote of the week:

What I will do for me this week...

To Do List

- ❑
- ❑
- ❑
- ❑
- ❑
- ❑

Thoughts....

Empowering Quote Of The Week

Quote of the week:

What I will do for me this week...

To Do List

- ☐
- ☐
- ☐
- ☐
- ☐
- ☐

Thoughts....

Empowering Quote Of The Week

Quote of the week:

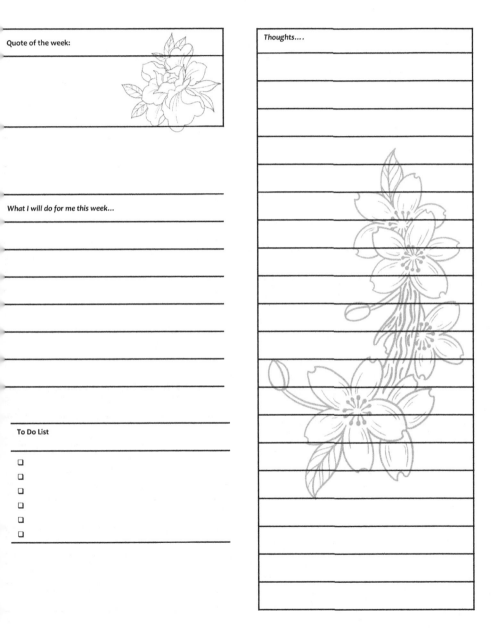

What I will do for me this week...

To Do List

- ☐
- ☐
- ☐
- ☐
- ☐
- ☐

Thoughts....

Empowering Quote Of The Week

Quote of the week:

What I will do for me this week...

To Do List

- ❑
- ❑
- ❑
- ❑
- ❑
- ❑

Thoughts....

Monthly Prompts

Monthly Gratitude
List what you are grateful for this month.

_____
_____
_____
_____
_____
_____

I am Learning…
What are you learning this month?

_____
_____
_____
_____
_____
_____

People in my Life
Who are you grateful for today and why?

_____
_____
_____
_____
_____
_____

Reflection
Write about the best part of your month.

_____
_____
_____
_____
_____
_____

Best Times of This Month

Date:

_____

What I saw:

Things I heard:

What I tasted:

My Feelings:

My Choices:

My Actions:

My Goals:

Overall thoughts of the month:

My Goals For This Month

Month _____

Describe Your Goal

_____

_____

_____

_____

Why I Want to Achieve This Goal

_____

_____

_____

Steps I Will Take To Achieve My Goal

1. _____

2. _____

3. _____

4. _____

KNOW YOUR WORTH, then add tax

My motivation for this month is:

_____

_____

I want to work on this because:

_____

_____

_____

_____

Reflections

_____

_____

_____

_____

_____

_____

_____

Today's Affirmation

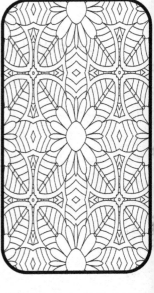

Empowering Quote Of The Week

Quote of the week:

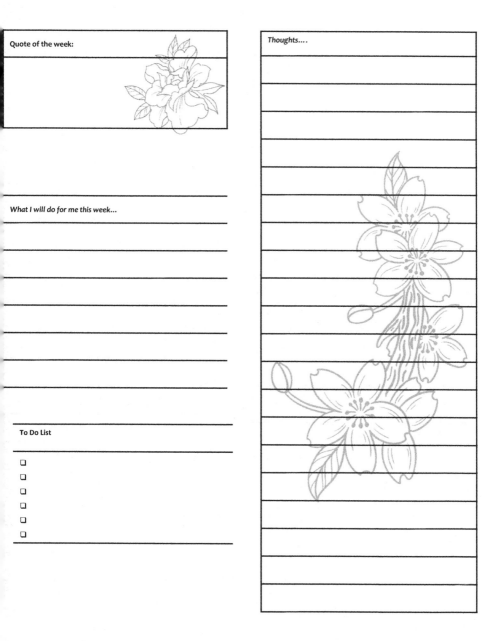

What I will do for me this week...

To Do List

- ☐
- ☐
- ☐
- ☐
- ☐
- ☐

Thoughts....

Empowering Quote Of The Week

Quote of the week:

What I will do for me this week...

To Do List

- ☐
- ☐
- ☐
- ☐
- ☐
- ☐

Thoughts....

Empowering Quote Of The Week

Quote of the week:

What I will do for me this week...

To Do List

- ☐
- ☐
- ☐
- ☐
- ☐
- ☐

Thoughts....

Empowering Quote Of The Week

Quote of the week:

What I will do for me this week...

To Do List

- ☐
- ☐
- ☐
- ☐
- ☐
- ☐

Thoughts... .

Monthly Prompts

Monthly Gratitude
List what you are grateful for this month.

_____
_____
_____
_____
_____
_____
_____

I am Learning...
What are you learning this month?

_____
_____
_____
_____
_____
_____
_____

People in my Life
Who are you grateful for today and why?

_____
_____
_____
_____
_____
_____
_____

Reflection
Write about the best part of your month.

_____
_____
_____
_____
_____
_____
_____

Best Times of This Month

Date: _____

What I saw:

Things I heard:

What I tasted:

My Feelings:

My Choices:

My Actions:

My Goals:

Overall thoughts of the month:

My Goals For This Month

Month _____

Describe Your Goal

_____

_____

_____

_____

Why I Want to Achieve This Goal

_____

_____

_____

Steps I Will Take To Achieve My Goal

1. _____

2. _____

3. _____

4. _____

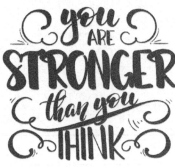

My motivation for this month is:

_____

_____

I want to work on this because:

_____

_____

_____

_____

Reflections

_____

_____

_____

_____

_____

_____

_____

Today's
Affirmation

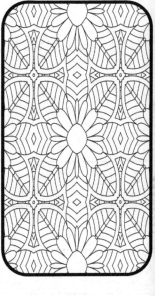

Empowering Quote Of The Week

Quote of the week:

What I will do for me this week...

To Do List

- ☐
- ☐
- ☐
- ☐
- ☐
- ☐

Thoughts....

Empowering Quote Of The Week

Quote of the week:

What I will do for me this week...

To Do List

- ❑
- ❑
- ❑
- ❑
- ❑
- ❑

Thoughts....

Empowering Quote Of The Week

Quote of the week:

What I will do for me this week...

To Do List

- ☐
- ☐
- ☐
- ☐
- ☐
- ☐

Thoughts....

Empowering Quote Of The Week

Quote of the week:

What I will do for me this week...

To Do List

- ☐
- ☐
- ☐
- ☐
- ☐
- ☐

Thoughts....

Monthly Prompts

Monthly Gratitude
List what you are
grateful for this month.

_____
_____
_____
_____
_____
_____
_____

I am Learning...
What are you learning
this month?

_____
_____
_____
_____
_____
_____

People in my Life
Who are you grateful for
today and why?

_____
_____
_____
_____
_____
_____

Reflection
Write about the best
part of your month.

_____
_____
_____
_____
_____

Best Times of This Month

Date:
_____

What I saw:

Things I heard:

What I tasted:

My Feelings:

My Choices:

My Actions:

My Goals:

Overall thoughts of the month:

My Goals For This Month

Month _____

Describe Your Goal

_____

_____

_____

_____

Why I Want to Achieve This Goal

_____

_____

_____

Steps I Will Take To Achieve My Goal

1. _____

2. _____

3. _____

4. _____

Motivation Keeps Me Movin'

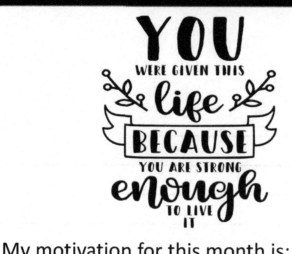

Today's
Affirmation

My motivation for this month is:

_____

_____

I want to work on this because:

_____

_____

_____

_____

Reflections

_____

_____

_____

_____

_____

_____

_____

_____

Empowering Quote Of The Week

Quote of the week:

What I will do for me this week...

To Do List

- ☐
- ☐
- ☐
- ☐
- ☐
- ☐

Thoughts....

Empowering Quote Of The Week

Quote of the week:

What I will do for me this week...

To Do List

- ☐
- ☐
- ☐
- ☐
- ☐
- ☐

Thoughts....

Empowering Quote Of The Week

Quote of the week:

What I will do for me this week...

To Do List

- ❏
- ❏
- ❏
- ❏
- ❏
- ❏

Thoughts....

Empowering Quote Of The Week

Quote of the week:

Thoughts….

What I will do for me this week...

To Do List

- ☐
- ☐
- ☐
- ☐
- ☐
- ☐

Monthly Prompts

Monthly Gratitude
List what you are grateful for this month.

_____
_____
_____
_____
_____
_____

I am Learning…
What are you learning this month?

_____
_____
_____
_____
_____

People in my Life
Who are you grateful for today and why?

_____
_____
_____
_____
_____

Reflection
Write about the best part of your month.

_____
_____
_____
_____
_____

Best Times of This Month

Date:
_____

What I saw:

Things I heard:

What I tasted:

My Feelings:

My Choices:

My Actions:

My Goals:

Overall thoughts of the month:

Notes

Notes

53415198R00070